Digest Alive
Lose Weight and Build a
Great Body, Naturally

Written by Acharya D Hargreaves

ISBN 978-0-6151-7046-6

This is a reference work.
It is not meant for diagnosis or treatment and it is not a substitute for
consultation with a licensed health care provider.

Cover art designed by Acharya D Hargreaves

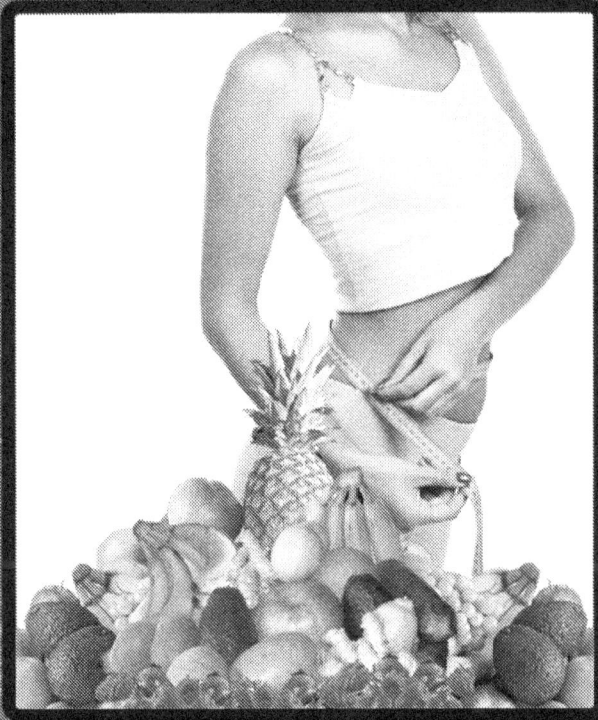

Digest Alive

Lose Weight and Build a Great Body Naturally

Acharya D Hargreaves

Our bodies always want to be balanced
Lets work with our bodies, not against them

3

Acknowledgments

I would like to say thank-you to my wonderful family who have inspired me in my many goals and desires to succeed in my life and who gave me inspiration in writing this small book.

I sincerely hope and desire that anyone who reads this book will get help from some of my suggestions in becoming fit, healthy and as slim as they desire.

Table of Contents

Introduction

Hello my name is Acharya D Hargreaves, Author of D*igest Alive The Natural Cure to Heartburn* and *Digest Alive Lose Weight and Build a Great Body Naturally*

I have always been underweight, I am about 6 feet tall with a thin body and tons of energy. I weigh about 135 pounds. I studied for months on how I could gain weight and I found out a lot about how to lose weight and what causes weight gain in people that are trying to lose it.

So this book is on how those of you that have too much weight can easily lose it and start living the life you dream of.

I am still looking for the answers for myself and someday I am sure I will find what I am looking for.

Chapter One

How stress causes weight gain

"Chronic stress and cortisol can contribute to weight gain" - Elizabeth Scott

Stress is one of the biggest factors that contribute to weight gain and obesity in many people today.

There are several ways stress can contribute to gaining unwanted weight and one of them is called the fight or flight response. When our bodies are under stress we activate the fight or flight response. It triggers in our bodies the release of different hormones such as adrenalin and cortisol.

These hormones speed the heart rate, slow digestion, shut down blood flow to major muscle groups and change various other autonomic nervous functions. This gives the body enough energy and strength to either fight or run away from danger.

It is our body's natural way of protecting itself. In today's stresses, we don't usually need to fight someone or run away to save ourselves.

Everyday, we have stressful times that we must face, like in traffic or during a stressful day at work. So, when we return home from our stressful environment, our bodies are ready to replenish themselves.

They need to return to their normal state by the relaxation response. If we don't let our bodies relax, then all the stress that is still in our bodies will start to cause damage.

When our bodies are under stress, the hormones corticotrophin and adrenalin are released. These hormones produce a reaction that stimulates the release of cortisol from the adrenal cortex.

Cortisol releases glucose into the bloodstream. When we are over stressed, the glucose releases an abundant amount of insulin into our body. Insulin is part of the endocrine system that is a fat storage hormone. This hormone overrides the stress signal from adrenalin to burn fat. The excess release of insulin gives the body the message to store fat in the abdomen and thighs.

The hormone cortisol can also contribute in other ways to weight gain such as metabolism and cravings.

Metabolism: When we are under stress, and our bodies starts to put out cortisol, this hormone can slow our metabolism, causing more weight gain than would normally happen. This also makes dieting more difficult.

Cravings: If our bodies are under a lot of stress, they can start to crave fattier, salty, sweet and sugary foods, also processed food and other things that are not as good for us. These foods are typically less healthy and lead to increased weight gain, because they make our bodies feel extra protection.

There are other ways our bodies put on fat from too much stress, like emotional eating, fast food and not enough exercise.

Emotional Eating: Emotional eating is an easy way to gain fat, because when we are angry, sad or frustrated, our bodies send out a signal that they need support. Our bodies then start to produce this hormone cortisol, which makes us crave unhealthy food so our bodies can feel more protected from all the stress.

The hormone cortisol, also releases an excess of nervous energy, which often can cause people to eat more than they normally would.

Fast Food: Eating fast food can also cause a lot of stress and abuse on our systems, especially, if we don't eat right and are in a hurry. The more stress which is in our life the more protection our bodies will feel they need and they will take action to balance themselves out. This means putting on more weight.

Not enough Exercise: Our bodies need a good amount of exercise everyday, to feel healthy and strong. If we don't get some exercise even a little every day our bodies will start to feel stress in the way we carry ourselves, in the way we sit and stand. Exercise is essential for keeping our bodies in shape, so that we don't have to work so hard to stay healthy.

Stress relief

Here are some things we can do to reduce the daily stress, so that our bodies don't have to work so hard and will not put on more fat than they need. To follow all of these suggestions may be too much if our day is a very busy one, but if we implement any one of these, our daily life will be more stress free.

Hot shower or Bath: Take a hot bath or shower in the evening after work is finished. Taking a hot shower or bath helps to relax all the muscles in our bodies, providing release of all the built up tension and excess adrenalin.

Massage: Getting a massage not only helps our bodies relax and release built up tensions and stress but they also help our bodies be more flexible and look younger. We can take a dry massage or an oil massage depending on what we are more comfortable with. Both are good.

Breathing deep: We can lie down on our backs and breathe deep, letting all our limbs rest and relax. While we are lying we can try to imagine the built up energy shooting out of us, through our fingers and toes. We can also put on some relaxing music. The key here is to breath deep and let all our limbs release the built up tension.

Yoga: We can do some yoga stretching to release our built up tension. Yoga is a form of exercise that will give us stress of our muscles but it's a different kind of stress that helps to promote healthy firmness of our joints and muscles. Yoga also has the ability to help center and calm the mind. This can be a great stress reliever.

Walking: Taking a long relaxing walk outside so that we can breathe the fresh air and release all the stored up energy.

John Gray says in his book *How to get what you want and want what you have:* Plants, trees and large bodies of water such as lakes and the ocean have a very wonderful ability to take our negative energy and stress and turn it into energy they can use to grow.

That is why we feel so refreshed whenever we go for a walk outside in a park or near a lake.

Our three bodies in one

"How to Become Right with the Physical Body and How to Make it Beautiful!" - *Dr Joshua David Stone*

Fantastic article about the beauty within, and taking care of our bodies. Each one of us have three bodies, we have

. A Physical body

. An Emotional body And

. A Spiritual body

All of these bodies need care.

All our bodies are connected and are part of a whole. If we neglect the care of one of them, then the others start to become neglected. So, by taking care of all three, we can become fully balanced and achieve success in anything we do.

When we are fully engaged in taking care of our bodily needs, such as keeping our bodies in good shape, exercising, eating right and living a stress free lifestyle.

Our emotional needs such as keeping good friendships, having a long and happy marriage, living with our loved ones and tolerating, forgiving and understanding others.

Finally our spiritual needs such as chanting gods name, reading Gods books, praying and giving praise to God and helping others that are less fortunate then us. We become most happy.

Our physical body

Our physical body is our outer body, flesh and bones. This is the body we work physically to build and to keep healthy. By keeping this body in shape and in health, we build our self-esteem, our self-confidence and our love for ourselves.

When we work hard to have a good physical body, it means that we are truly grateful for our body. By keeping it in shape, in optimal health and appearance we build our love and appreciation for ourselves.

We also build an image that is appreciated by others. When we work hard to create a good image of our outer appearance, others see it and think highly about us.

They see that we are achievers, that we are someone special and because of this more and more people will want to be around us, or with us. They will want to listen to us. This creates self-confidence in ourselves, which helps our other bodies as well.

Our emotional body

Our emotional body is our second body. This body is like our subtle body. It is what deals with our emotions. Having a satisfied emotional body is very essential, because without our emotional body in balance, our emotions start to wreck havoc on our physical body.

Our emotions are what drive us to do the things we do to our physical body. Without a balanced emotional state, our emotions would start to tell us things that would not benefit our body, such as "You're not strong enough to exercise everyday why don't you skip it today. Tomorrow you can try again" or "I don't care about your health right now, I'm sad and I need support why don't you eat something, so I can feel better."

Our emotional body loves attention and when we satisfy it with good attention then it becomes pleased and is willing to co-operate with our other bodies.

Our spiritual body

Our spiritual body is our soul. Our soul is our body which is connected with God or the universe. By helping our soul to become more in tune with God or the universe, we become more happy ourselves.

The soul controls our love, joy and happiness that we feel everytime we help someone, everytime we do a good deed or give our love and support. Every time we praise God or give thanks to the universe, our soul becomes happier.

Our spiritual body is the life giving force within ourselves. Without it, we would not be able to move, think, feel, or do anything for that matter. The soul is what gives us life.

How to keep all three healthy

Our physical body

We need to keep our physical body fit, strong, and healthy by doing daily exercises, by eating right and by doing our best to live a stress free lifestyle. If we can achieve these things, our physical body will be in top shape. We will feel full of life, energy, vigor, strength and confidence.

Our emotional body will thank us for our efforts because from having, a well toned and healthy body, we create good remarks and admiration from others. We also have good sex appeal. Our emotional body loves these things, so by keeping our physical body healthy we start to help our emotional body as well.

There are many exercises, that can help to create a great figure, and I have listed a few in the second chapter that will greatly help in creating the figure desire most.

Our emotional body

We need to keep our emotional body healthy by keeping good relationships and fixing broken ones.

If we keep hold of old broken relationships and don't try to fix them, either by healing the relationship or by forgiving and then forgetting the relationship then our emotional body still feels hurt, and the hurt can cause other problems.

Another thing about our emotional body is that it keeps thousands upon thousands of situations and thoughts inside itself. If any of these thoughts or situations are not fulfilled or completed then we are renting rent-free space in our brain for those hurtful or unfulfilled things.

If we can complete those things or forgive and forget, we can open our emotional body to better and greater things to come.

One way to help our emotional body is by talking to ourself in a mirror. This may sound funny at first but it is a very good way of helping our emotional body in its health. We can start out by asking our self

"How are you today?"

and

"It is good to see you again".

Then we can start by saying

"I would like to complement you today on..."

We then start to list all the things that we have accomplished today. They can be very little things like going for a walk, or chewing our food properly so that our digestion will work better, or that we made a step towards a better relationship with someone, or that we are doing more exercise, or we are completing one of our goals.

Our emotional body loves hearing all these praises and it will thank us afterwards by giving us a happy and satisfied feeling.

After we are finished talking to our emotional body, we can tell ourself in the mirror that we love ourself. Having a healthy respect for our self is very important.

Saying this to ourself, helps a great deal in balancing our bodies, because many times we may feel that our life is missing love, or friendship, or we may be unsatisfied with our physical body and because of that unsatisfied feeling, our emotional body is affected.

However, when we tell ourself that we care and we do love ourself our emotional body becomes happier and is then more willing to listen to our needs.

Our spiritual body

We can keep our spiritual body happy by giving in charity to others in need, by being kind and humble to others, by praising God or the universe, by setting an example for others to follow.

Anything that we can do that will help others in living better, in feeling better and in learning more about God or the universe makes the soul happier. Our souls are happiest when they are in tune with God or the universe. So, by doing acts of kindness and charity to the less fortunate ones, we can further our progress towards the greater good.

If we can practice on a daily basis, be kind to everyone, be humble to others, and learn to forgive and forget, our souls will develop a great happiness, which will help us to become balanced in all three of our bodies.

Visualization

"In order to change the printout of the body, we must learn to rewrite the software of the mind." – Deepak Chopra, M.D.

Visualization is also a very important part of helping our bodies become balanced. By visualizing on a daily basis that we are healthy, that we have a really great body and that we are feeling strong and vigorous, can greatly help our emotional bodies in their processes of turning our physical bodies into what we desire.

Visualizing is kind of like the programming we can do to our emotional bodies. Once our emotional bodies are happy and believe that we are what we have been visualizing, they will work things out so that our physical bodies achieve the images we have planted into our emotional bodies minds.

So, we should start visualizing that we are beautiful people, that we are strong, healthy, active individuals. The only thing that can come from this exercise is good. So we have nothing to lose by trying it out. Continually telling ourselves that we are beautiful, that we are strong and healthy, that we are slim and fit will start to create a happy feeling inside us whenever we look at ourselves in the mirror.

Some people may think it is somewhat crazy if we talk to ourselves in the mirror, and if so we should do it when we are alone. Married couples should get each other involved.

Chapter Two

Losing weight naturally

The most important thing to know is that there is no easy way to lose weight, such as taking a magic pill or something. Losing weight takes patience and endurance, but it can be easily achieved if we are determined.

Our bodies always want to be balanced; However, when we put stress on our bodies, like not enough exercise, not eating properly and doing things that weaken our bodies, like smoking, drinking and over eating junk food, our bodies compensate by putting more fat and weight on, so that we feel more balanced to take all the abuse.

Our bodies cannot and will not lose weight unless they feel as though they are unbalanced and need to balance themselves out by losing weight. To do this we must help our bodies get back to their original balanced state.

First off, the best way to start out is to find something we like doing which is physical that will make us break a sweat after working at it for a while.

We should start a daily routine doing an exercise that we enjoy like swimming, biking, horseback riding, walking, dancing, rope jumping, jogging, hiking, or anything else that can cause us to break a sweat.

Playing with children is also a good way to break a sweat. This not only helps to lose weight but it also helps create a wonderful bond between mother or father and child. We should only do our exercise until we break a sweat, then stop.

If we repeat this every day, we will see some astonishing results. When we are exercising at something we enjoy doing, it becomes so much easier to keep it up everyday as opposed to doing something for the sake of reducing weight only. If there is no fun in what we are doing, we will stop eventually and our bodies will go back into their states of distress.

When our bodies reach the sweating point, they are letting us know that we are burning fat and calories. Therefore, that means we are losing weight.

However, doing this is not enough alone. If we are still abusing our bodies and trying to lose weight at the same time, our bodies will try to compensate by putting on even more weight to replace the weight it just lost.

The second part to helping our bodies achieve their natural state is to start eating properly and building a good digestion so that our bodies will not be compensating for any extra abuse.

Some people eat excessively fast. They do not chew their food. Also they eat mostly indigestible foods that are extremely low in nutrients. These things are what cause a lot of stress on our digestive system.

That is why our bodies gain extra fat to support all that extra abuse. Next we will discuss digestive health and how we can lose weight and build a great looking body by toning our bodies with specific exercises. Doing the toning exercises is extra.

We should however do some kind of exercise we love doing everyday, something that gives us joy. That type of exercise is essential. We are not required to practice the toning exercises to lose weight, although they will defiantly help us to build a fantastic body.

Digestive Health

To help take care of the balancing of our bodies we should start getting our digestion in order. Having a healthy, working digestion will immensely improve our bodies balancing and will help us to lose weight as well.

Digestive health is very important in keeping a healthy body. Having a healthy digestion is basically the key ingredient in having the best health. So, to build a good digestion we must start off with these simple steps. We should try to do them everyday. This will greatly increase our digestive strength and improve our immune system, as well.

My first book **Digest Alive The Natural Cure to Heartburn** gives a more in depth discussion of how to improve our overall digestion and a list of herbs, fruits and vegetables that help increase digestive absorption

First off, we must remember to chew our food until it is almost liquid. That will greatly help in our digestion, since our saliva will have adequately

performed the beginning digestive process.
It may not sound so appealing but this simple task
will improve things immensely.

Remember not to eat too much. Overeating will
cause fermentation and gas to start to build up
inside the stomach. Also, that would cause
unnecessary weight gain.

Our stomachs only have a certain amount of
hydrochloric acid and digestive enzymes each time
that we eat. So if we have too much food in our
stomachs, the food will not be digested properly
and will start to ferment. So, we need to eat only
until we feel almost full. Then stop.

A good way to measure is to eat only until we have
our first or second burp. Our bodies are telling us
something. We need to listen to them and stop
when we burp.

We should stop eating during bedtime hours.
Around 8:00 or 9:00 PM our stomachs stop
performing their digestion and our bodies start
getting everything ready for resting and recovery
for the next day.

Food eaten during bedtime hours mostly sits in our
stomachs. It sabotages our digestive enzymes for
the next day and gives us bad breath in the
morning. Eating on a regular time table or schedule

helps as well. It will help to maintain a balanced digestion.

The digestion in our bodies is like the element of fire. If we think of the stomach as our furnace, then to increase digestion, we must make more heat.

One of the best ways to intensify a fire is to feed it oxygen. If we can do some exercise before we eat then our digestion will improve and our bodies will be able to digest the food better.

Jogging, swimming, walking all do the job. Exercise builds appetite and the higher temperatures of a well-oxygenated body achieve more efficient combustion. If exercising is not convenient, doing 5 minutes of deep breathing just before eating also helps to increase digestion for proper assimilation.

Also, relaxing while we eat is a great way to help our digestions in their process. Siting down in a comfortable place where we can enjoy our food as much as possible. That way, our bodies are not under any kind of stress and can accept the food that is put into them more easily.

Being in a stressful state while we eat is not good. So we should do our best to be in a happy state of mind while we eat. One of the best ways of reducing stress is to breath deep three times and then we can ask our minds a positive question that has nothing to do with what we were thinking about.

Physiologists say that the brain can only think of one thing at a time, and if we can replace the painful or negative thought with a more positive thought then our pain or stress will instantly go away.

We should try to think positively while we are eating. Thinking positively all day, actually, is great. But it takes some time to get used to thinking this way. Ok. So, here we go.

Number one: We chew our food until it is almost liquid.

Number two: Remember not to eat too much. We can use our first or second burps as a guideline.

Number three: No eating during bedtime hours. The stomach stops performing its digestion at this time and our bodies start getting everything ready for resting and recovery for the next day.

Number four: Relax, for the best effect. We should be in a relaxed, calm state for our digestion to have its best effect.

Dieting

Dieting is one way we gain weight. Most people think that dieting helps us to lose weight but this is not the case.

When we start a diet and reduce our food intake, our bodies start to think that we are stranded on a desert island and they turn on our alert system. Because we are dieting, our bodies get the impression that food is scarce and therefore they start to slow down our metabolism so our bodies are able to get the best use of the small amount of food they are receiving.

When our bodies start to slow down our metabolism, we start to gain weight from the small amounts of food we consume. If our bodies had a high rate of metabolism then we would burn most of our nutrients as energy, but with a slow metabolism our bodies have a much slower burn rate.

Our bodies are designed to hold on to fat from the food we eat so we have enough protection and energy stored for a longer period of time. If our bodies are thinking that we will need to have food for later because we are stranded on a desert island, then our bodies will try to store the fat for later use when we might need it the most.

Our bodies use the stored up fat for energy by breaking it down with enzymes which release glycerol and fatty acids which get put into the bloodstream.

When our bodies need energy they use the fatty acids and send them to the mitochondria of the cell that needs the extra energy. The mitochondria are places where our bodies can extract the energy they need from the fat and carbohydrates we consume.

The Good, The Bad and The Ugly Fats

We can relax knowing that most fats are very healthy and vital to our overall health.

Many people believe that any kind of fat is bad for the body, that is why we have so many products which advertise less fat or non fat, but in actuality our bodies can't live without fat. Good fat is absolutely essential for good health, without it we would shrivel up and die.

Some of the good fats are non-saturated fats such as polyunsaturated, mono-unsaturated and surprisingly saturated fats. These types of fats or oils have many good uses for our bodies.

Saturated fat is a very good form of fat for our bodies. It make up at least 50% of our cell membranes, which helps keep our cells strong. It helps keep our bones strong by helping calcium to be effectively incorporated into our skeletal structure.

It lowers the risk of heart disease. It helps protect

the liver from alcohol and other toxins which may be harmful. It helps the immune system and much more.

There is an amazing article "The Truth About Saturated Fat" on a website called "The Best Natural Health Information and Newsletter." There we can find out more info on saturated fats as well as other fats.

The web address is **http://www.mercola.com**

Polyunsaturated fat includes the omega 3 and omega 6 fatty acids. Which our bodies greatly need because these essential fatty acids our bodies can not produce on their own. We need to get them from other sources.

We can find polyunsaturated fats in many vegetable oils like safflower oil, corn oil, sunflower oil, flax seed oil, hemp oil, pumpkin seeds, walnuts and soybeans.

Mono-unsaturated fats are some of the healthiest types of fats we can eat. They typically are high in vitamin e and anti-oxidant properties.

We can find mono-unsaturated fats in olive oil, rapeseed oil, hazelnuts, almonds, Brazil nuts, cashews, avocado, sesame seeds and pumpkin seeds.

Trans fats are the bad fats that turn ugly, these are the fats we all will want to avoid. Trans fats are artery clogging fats, they can increase bad cholesterol, type 2 diabetes, heart disease and many other kinds of illness.

Trans fats are found in foods like margarine, shortening, french fries, fried chicken, dough nuts as well as other extra processed foods.

If we make our own fried foods or dough nuts with a better oil then we can eat them without worry.

But the bottom line here is that most fats today are healthy for our bodies, so trying to eat only non fat foods to stay thin is actually a bad idea if we want to lose weight.

Our body's metabolism

Our bodies metabolic rates are controlled by our thyroid glands. Our thyroid glands are found just below our Adam's apples, even women have Adam's apples, just very small ones.

Our thyroid glands control how quickly our bodies burn energy, make proteins and how sensitive our bodies are to other hormones. Our thyroid glands are also responsible for our metabolism, how fast or how slow our bodies burn fats and carbohydrates.

If our bodies have an under active thyroid or Hypothyroidism, then our thyroid glands will produce less thyroid hormones which in turn slow down our metabolic rate. If our bodies have a slow metabolic rate we start to store fat.

The best way to avoid getting Hypothyroidism is to get enough iodine in the food we eat. Taking kelp or seaweed in or on our food is an excellent way to get the iodine we need for helping our thyroids to stay healthy and balanced.

By having a balanced thyroid our bodies will then

40

balance our metabolism which in turn will help keep us thin, healthy and fit.

Simple toning exercises

If we want to create, a fit-looking, strong body with some nice stomach muscles or a great looking butt or thighs. What we need to do is tone our muscles.

Since we want to lose weight, we do not want to put on any more weight by building more muscle. So what we are going to do is tone the muscle we already have, that way we do not gain any muscle fat but still get great looking muscles.

Here are some very simple toning exercises that anyone can do to tone different parts of their body.

Firmer Breasts or Pectoral muscles

Images A. B. C. for first exercise and D. E. for second exercise, in exercise diagrams

First exercise: This is a simple yoga exercise in which we sit cross-legged with our arms at our sides. We take three deep breaths to relax our body and then we clasp our hands behind us and lift our arms up keeping them as straight and as high as we can. We keep our back straight and feel the tightening in our pectoral or Brest muscles.

We should only raise the arms as far as we can without too much pain, there should be a small tightening, stretching feeling in the pectoral or breast muscles. We keep this pose for a count of 10 and then lower our arms towards the ground, repeat three more times.

Second exercise: We can also do push-ups to tighten and tone our breasts or pectoral muscles. We place our hands shoulder width apart on the floor. Then we balance on our hands and the balls of our feet so our body forms a straight line.

Now we bend our elbows and our lower body half or all the way to the floor and hold for 5 seconds, then press back up to the starting position. Work towards the count of 30.

The more we can do these the better, but just start out with three in a row then rest and repeat twice more. If we go half-way to the floor, it is easier then all the way since we do not have as much gravity to push up against.

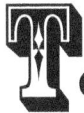

Toning your Abdominals or Abs

Images F. G. for first exercise and H. I. J. K. L. M. N. O. for second exercise, in exercise diagrams

First exercise: We lie with our back flat against the floor, with both legs straight.

We place our hands behind our heads in gentle support. We don't hold or lift our heads up or interlace our fingers together either.

Now we slowly lift our shoulders off the floor, using the strength of our abdominal muscles until we are sitting upright.

43

We should breathe out as we lift up, and then breathe in as we slowly lower our shoulders back to the floor in to the starting position. Repeat this exercise fifteen times. Do five times then take a rest and repeat twice more.

This was the fast version, we can also do a slower abdominal or abs exercise that has the same effect.

Second exercise: We sit up straight with our legs outstretched, then we reach towards our toes and touch our toes or ankles.

Now we slowly sit back up and grasp our thighs firmly with our hands, then we start to lower our upper body down to the floor as slowly as we can, keeping our legs straight and holding firmly onto our thighs for support, We use our abdominal muscles as much as possible to slow our decent.

Once we reach the floor, we should immediately start to bend our legs towards our chests. Once our legs are in a 90 degree angle, we straighten them up fully towards the ceiling and then start to lower them towards the floor keeping them straight.

Next we use our lower abdominal muscles as much as possible to slow the decent of our legs to the floor.

Once our legs are again in a straight position against the floor we can start to raise our upper body to the sitting position, we do this as slowly as we can, using our abdominal muscles to slow our ascent. We repeat three more times and take a rest. Then repeat the whole process again.

Thigh and Buttocks Toning exercises

Images P. Q. R. for this exercise, in exercise diagrams

First exercise: We stand up straight, with our knees slightly bent and with our feet hip distance apart with toes pointing forward. We breathe in as we squat down.

We should keep our shoulders and back straight as we complete this exercise. Now we bend our elbows and hold both arms in a boxer position, fists out in front.

We slowly start to bend our knees lowering our butts towards the floor. When we reach the point that our knees are in a 90-degree bend or our thighs are parallel to the ground, we hold this position for a count of five.

Balancing our bodies weight by pressing our weight through our heels, not our toes. Also we keep our knees over our ankles, not past our toes.

Our butts should be sticking outwards and our backs and shoulders should be straight, it is like sitting in a chair. If we want this exercise to be harder, we can lower our bodies past the sitting position.

We breathe out as we stand back up, squeezing our butt muscles.

Repeat exercise fifteen times

Organically Grown

Eating healthy, nutritious food is the best way to increase our overall health. Eating foods that contain high amounts of digestive enzymes in them helps to keep our digestion healthy and strong.

Most organic vegetables and fruits are the best since they were grown without any harmful pesticides. Fruits and vegetables very easily absorb pesticides, and the harmful chemicals are then stored in the skin of the vegetables or fruits.

Over time eating a lot of vegetables or fruits that are not organic can have bad affects on our health. The accumulation of the poisons from all the vegetables or fruits can start to cause illness and affect our digestion and immune systems.

If there is a farmer's market nearby they would probably have a good amount of organically grown vegetables or fruits we could buy at reasonable prices.

Buying organically grown may be more expensive but it is worth it. Making sure our health is at its peak is the most important in goal life, otherwise our life is usually a big pain!

Most meat will put on fat, and if our digestive systems are not working properly then eating meat, will defiantly have a bad affect on our digestion.

Vegetarianism or vegan are becoming very popular these days and even many celebrities are vegetarian or vegan. Most people are now discovering that the vegetarian lifestyle they lead, the healthier they are.

Weight loss Fruits

Eating lots of fruits are a great way to lose weight. We should never eat only fruits, because we would lose weight too quickly, but having a good amount of fruits in our diets is very beneficial to our weight loss.

Fruits are mostly made of water, so when we eat fruits we get vitamins and minerals as well as a satisfied full feeling, fruits though don't put on much weight when we eat them. They are mostly water and because of this they get dispelled out of our bodies very quickly.

There was a study done by the *American Journal of Clinical Nutrition* on June 22, 2007

The patients who reduce their dietary energy density by eating fruits and vegetables, and limiting fat intake loss a third more weight at 6 months compared to the patients who only decreased their fat intake.

This means the patients eating fruit and vegetables with their regular meals were able to lose weight faster then the ones that only reduced how much food or fat they ate.

So having good amounts of fruits and vegetables daily will help greatly in our weight loss. We can eat two or three servings a day of fruit, which means an apple is one serving a pear is another and orange is another.

Fruits and vegetables have many great benefits. One of them is fiber. Fiber goes hand in hand with healthy eating and losing weight.

Fiber, is a sugar-like substance that comes in thousands of forms. Eating the whole fruit or vegetable is actually better then just drinking the fruit or vegetable juice because we get to use the fiber in our bodies. Every vegetable and fruit has some fiber.

There are two major types of fiber in every fruit or vegetable. Insoluble and soluble. The insoluble fiber helps our bodies to have better waste evacuation because the bacteria in the lower bowel or colon do not break down this type of fiber.

Soluble fiber is used as a food source by the beneficial and colon bacteria. These beneficial bacteria then create the nutrition needed by the cells lining the colon.

Exercise diagrams

A

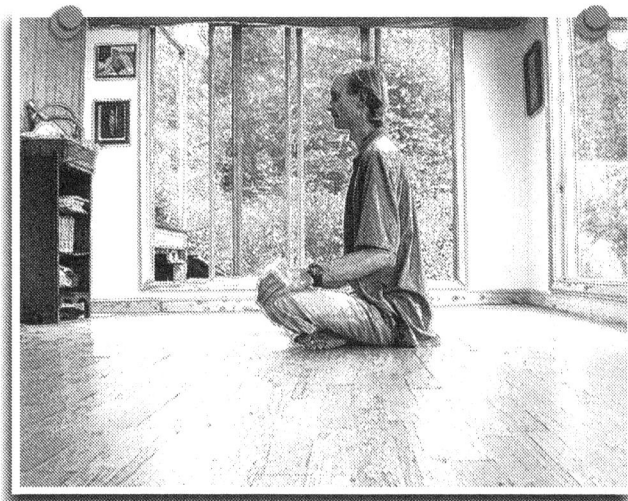

B

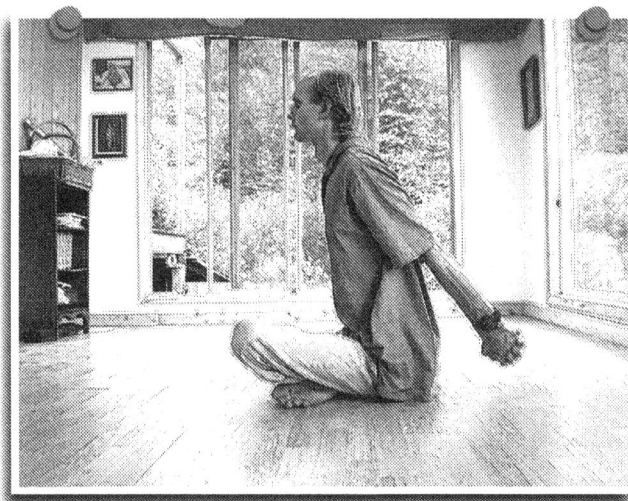

C

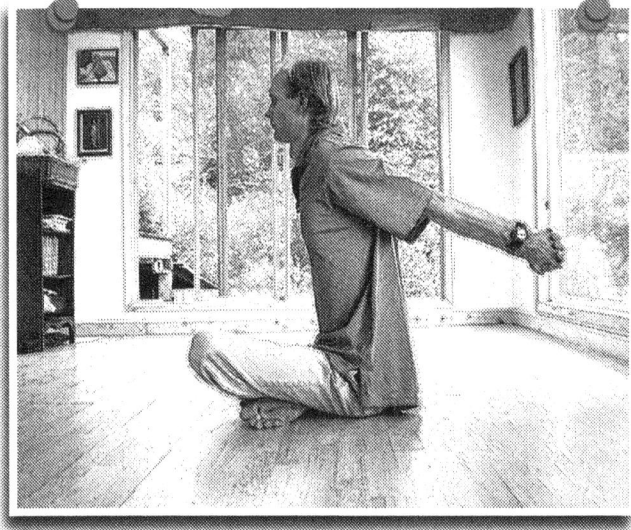

D

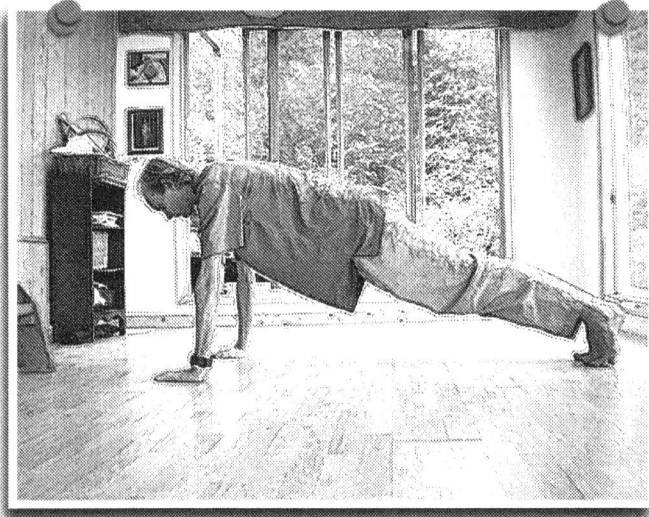

52

E

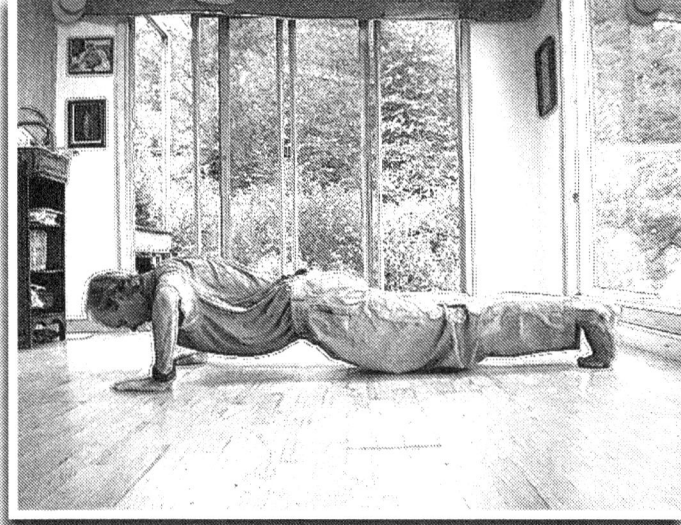

F

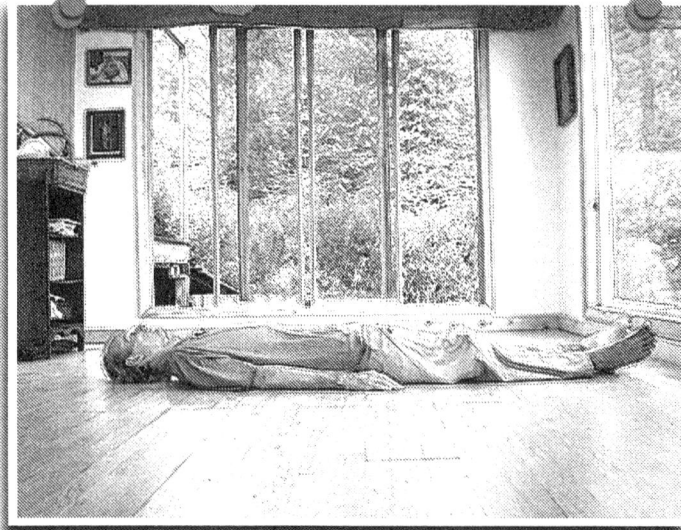

53

G

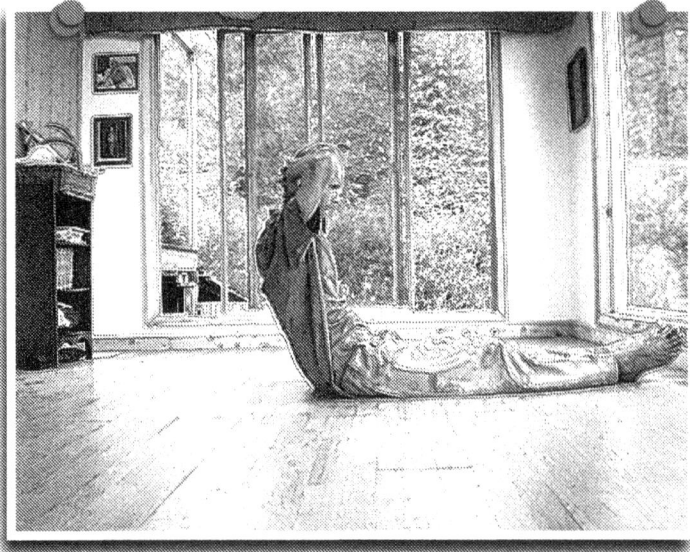

H

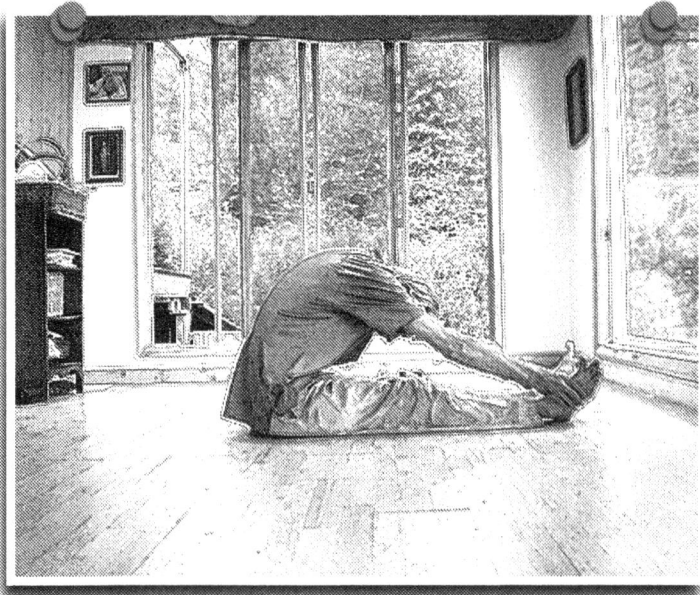

54

I

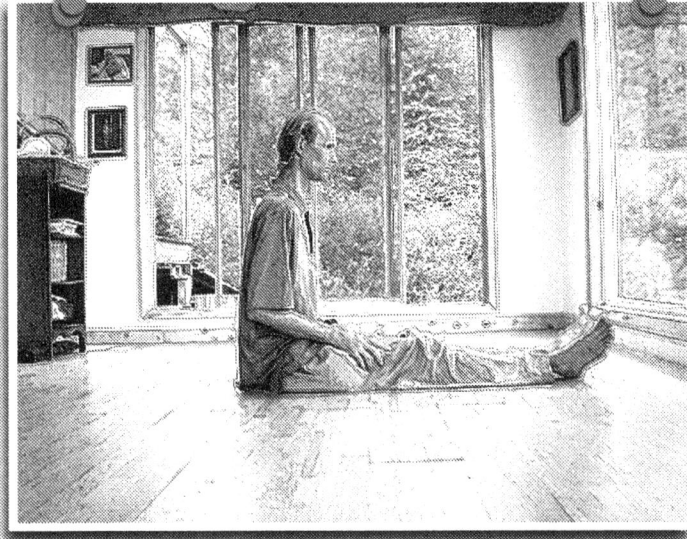

J

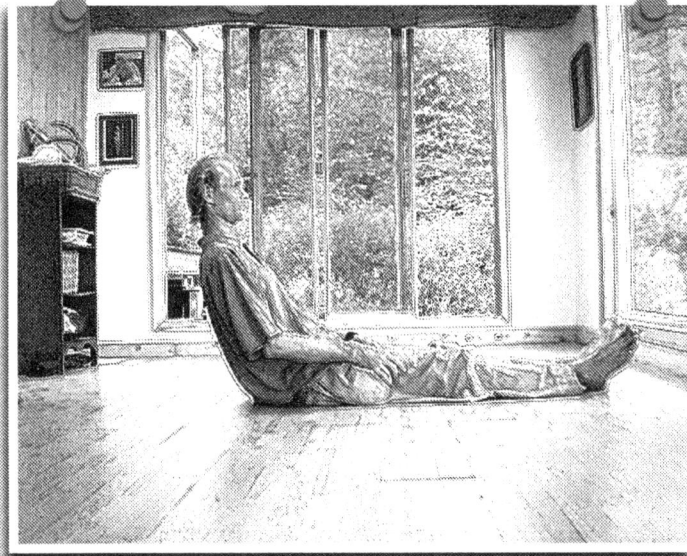

55

K

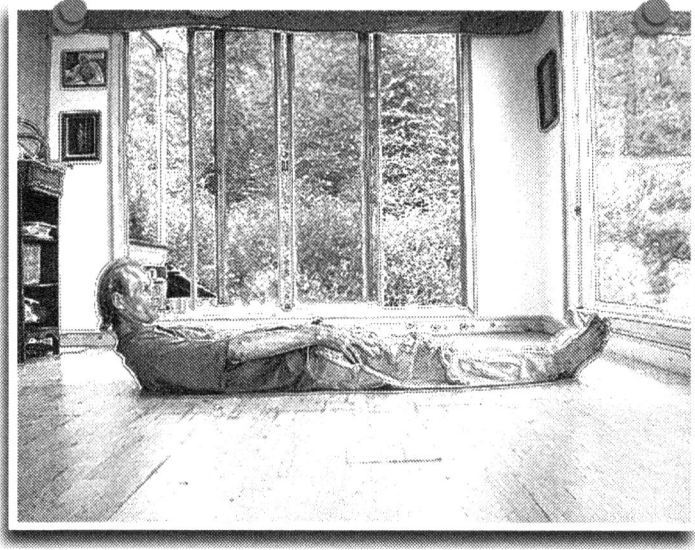

L

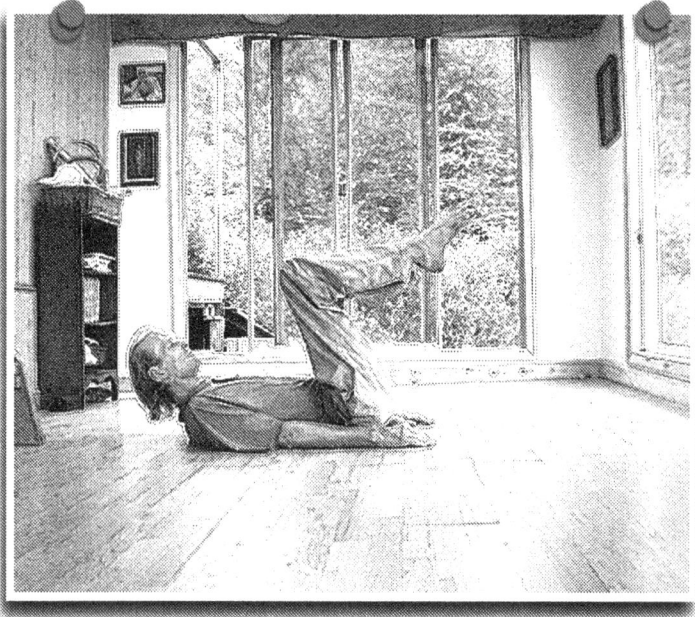

56

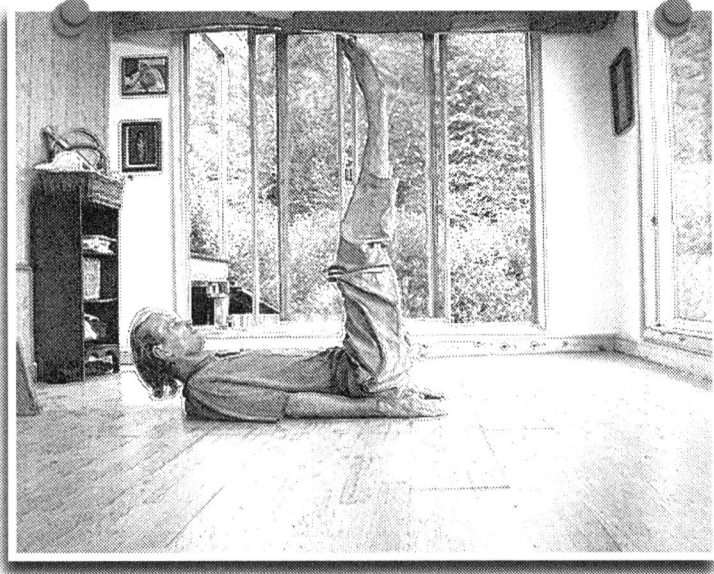

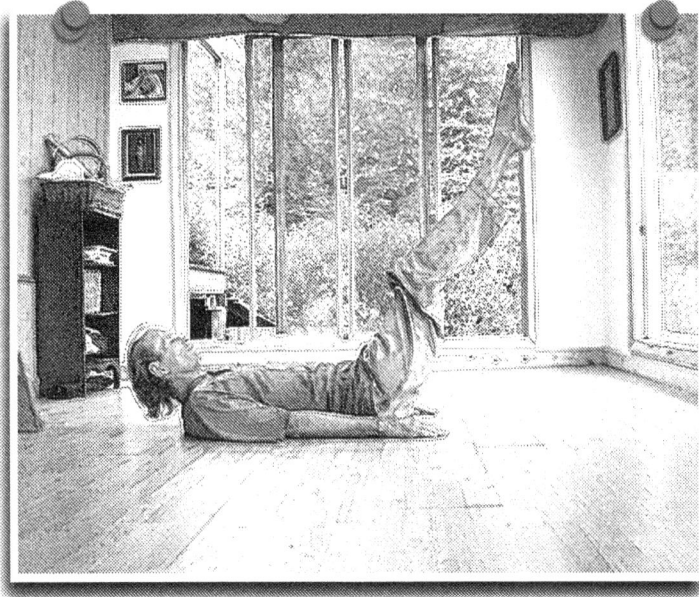

O

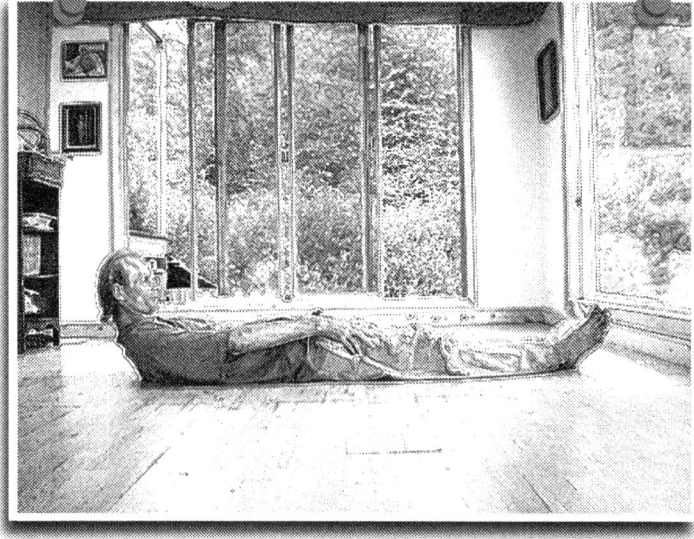

P

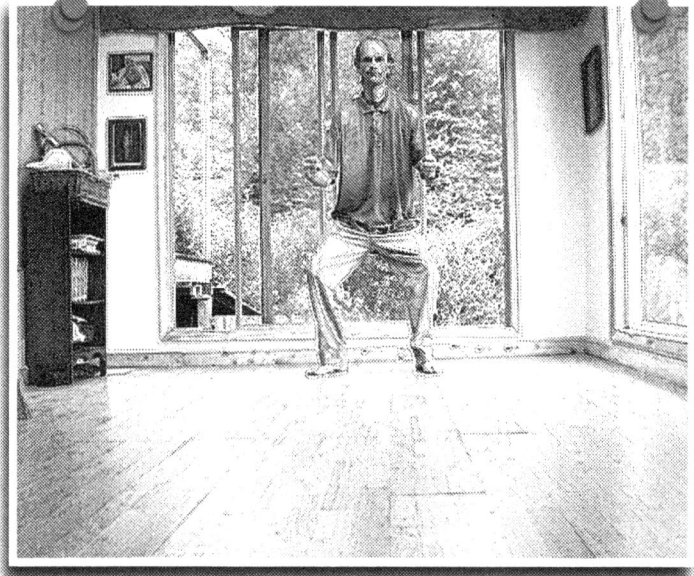

58

Q

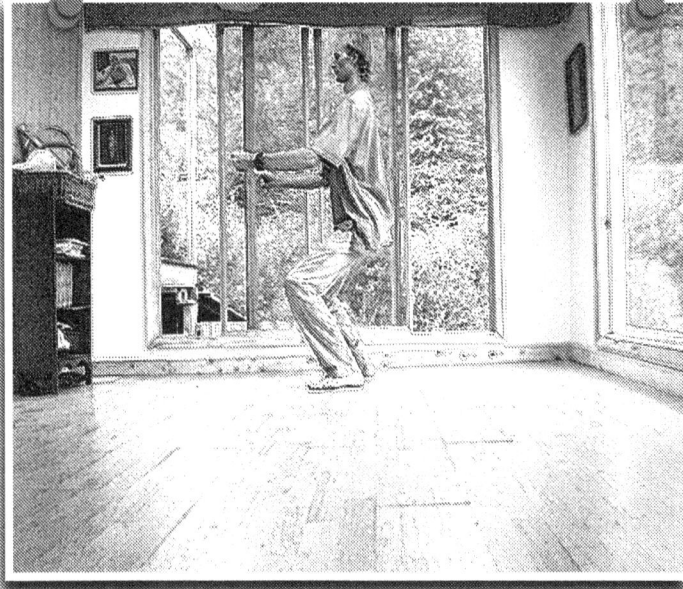

R

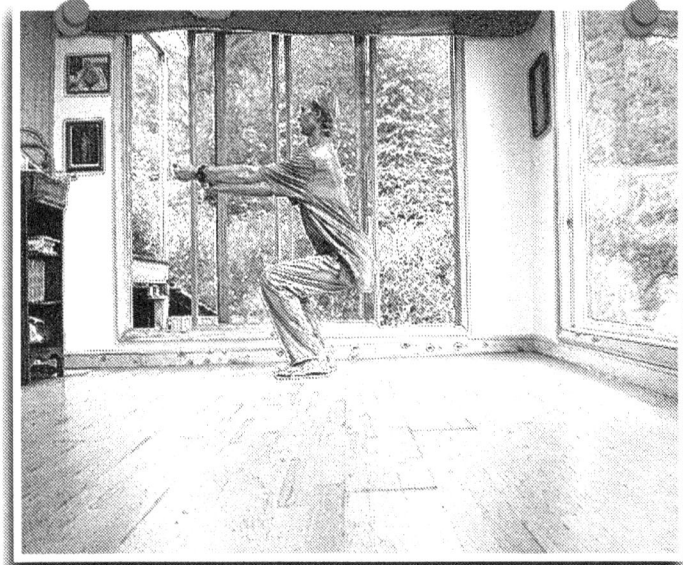

59

Summary

So the basic idea behind losing weight and keeping it off is to make sure our bodies are balanced by eating right, doing some kind of exercise that we enjoy so we don't quit exercising, doing our best to keep stress out of our lives by allowing our bodies to regenerate themselves after a stressful day at home or work and visualizing ourselves as beautiful, confident, positive, slim and fit individuals.

If we can accomplish these things in our lifetime, then we will achieve our desired image. We will lose weight and build a great body.

Reference directory

Deepak Chopra, M.D. - "In order to change the printout of the body, we must learn to rewrite the software of the mind."

Dr. Ferdowsian, MD, MPH, an internist preventative medicine and public health specialist and director of the Washington Center for Clinical Research.

Dr. John Gray, Author of *How to get what you want and want what you have*

Dr. Joseph Mercola, Author of *Take Control of Your Health*

Dr Joshua David Stone - "How to Become Right with the Physical Body and How to Make it Beautiful!"

Elizabeth Scott - "Chronic stress and cortisol can contribute to weight gain"

Frank W. Jackson MD, "losing weight, healthy eating, and fiber"

Gloria Tsang, R.D., is the chief editor for HealthCastle.com, a one-stop site for reliable nutrition information and tips

Linda Mackenzie C.H.T., Ph.D. - "How Does Visualization Work?"

Glossary of Terms

Adrenal cortex Maintains the stress response through the production of mineralocorticoids, glucocorticoids, aldosterone and cortisol.

Corticotrophin is a hormone produced by the anterior pituitary gland that stimulates the adrenal cortex.

Cortisol is an adrenal cortex hormone that is active in carbohydrate and protein metabolism.

Fight or flight response For example if a grazing gazelle is peacefully eating and it suddenly sees a lion run at it for a kill. The body initiates the fight or flight response.

Hormone Is a chemical signal from one cell to another cell.

Hypothyroidism is an under active thyroid gland, resulting from insufficient production of thyroid hormones.

Insulin Is a polypeptide hormone that regulates carbohydrate metabolism.

Organelle is a specialized part of a cell.

Mineralocorticoids and Glucocorticoids Are a class of steroid hormones, they influence the salt and water metabolism in the body.

Mitochondria is an organelle containing enzymes responsible for producing energy.

Pituitary gland is the master gland of the endocrine system, located at the base of the brain.

The endocrine system Is a control system of ductless glands that secrete chemical signals called hormones that circulate within the body via the bloodstream.

DISCLAIMER:

The purpose of this document is to provide general information. I personally believe in the information of this document because it helped me to cure my conditions, but this document is not a substitute for consultation with a physician. Statements contained herein have not been evaluated by the Food and Drug Administration. Use this information and if you are benefiting, please offer thanks and prayers to God, the source of knowledge. Moderation is a sign of wisdom and excess of anything, even water, can be dangerous.

www.ingramcontent.com/pod-product-compliance
Lightning Source LLC
Chambersburg PA
CBHW022131280326
41933CB00007B/637